I WISH I COULD(N'T)
CARE LESS

PATRICIA OGILVIE

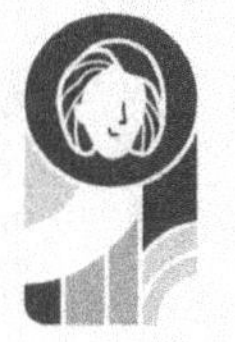

Box 253,
Alberta Beach, Alberta, Canada T0E 0A0
Modern Second Edition 2024
ISBN-13: 978-1979966269
ISBN-10: 1979966265

To my parents

CONTENTS

INTRODUCTION

Hello and welcome! First, you're entitled to an explanation about this book title:

People say they could care less when, logically, they mean they *couldn't* care less.

(The following grammatical definition is provided by Mignon Fogarty, Grammar Girl.)

The phrase "I couldn't care less" originated in Britain and made its way to the United States in the 1950s. The phrase "I could care less" appeared in the US about a decade later.

In 1990, Harvard professor and language writer Stephen Pinker argued that the way most people say could care less—the way they emphasize the words—implies they are being ironic or sarcastic.

Other linguists have argued that the type of sound at

the end of "couldn't" is naturally dropped by sloppy or slurring speakers.

Regardless of the reason people say they could care less, it is one of the more common language peeves because of its illogical nature. To say you could care less means you have a bit of caring left, which is not what I intend here. What I intend is to show you that when you care about what others think or say about you gets in the way of you living a fun, peaceful life, you should be able to state with bold confidence, "I couldn't care less!"

The proper "couldn't care less" is still the dominant form in print, but "could care less" has been steadily gaining ground since its appearance in the 1960s.

WHY DID I INCLUDE BOTH AND WHICH IS RIGHT?

If you care about what others think or say about you and that belief gets in the way of you living a fun, peaceful life, you should be able to proclaim with confidence, "I couldn't care less!" Another way to say it is simply, "I don't care!"

I titled this with both phrases because "could care less" is so common and I didn't want my reader, maybe you, to feel left out if you use one over the other. And now, just for fun, here's an example from the TV show *Psych*:

Juliet O'Hara: Guess what today is.

Carlton Lassiter: It's not one of those touchy-feely holidays invented by card companies to goad me into buying a present for someone I couldn't care less about, is it?

— - MAGGIE LAWSON PLAYING O'HARA
AND TIMOTHY OMUNDSON PLAYING
LASSITER

Now that that's cleared up, what you will find in this book are mega stories about (particularly) my experiences of caring too much about what other people think.

Sometimes that belief completely froze me. I often found myself stuck, unable to make decisions or move forward in building relationships. This was especially true when it came to social media, which I talk about here.

You will also find a lot of suggestions and solutions how to beat the beast. So now, let's get started handling how to care less and live better.

I know what you're thinking. Yeah right. I care too much about what people think. I've always done that. And now you're going to tell me I can stop? You're going to tell me grab my teddy bear, turn around and walk away?

Listen, you tell me, what do people who couldn't care less do? How do they think and would they walk away? Of course, they would! So why not you?

GRAB YOUR TEDDY BEAR (OR ANY COMFORT ITEM) AND WALK AWAY

All I want you to do is find some good reason to turn around and walk away without feeling bad. I want you to begin to feel better about who you are. And I wish you to begin to feel happier and less sad when you get into a deep mental frenzy thinking someone is talking about you, thinking about you, or blatantly disliking you. Eventually I would love to see you take up your own cause and say out loud – I really don't care what you think! The content here is simple, brief and your opportunity to be better equipped to cope with how you think about yourself. Let's go.

To begin, here's the story I remember and realized how it affected me through and through. Here is why I felt and mostly still feel that I care about what people say and do, way too much. And the reason is because I am afraid that if I don't care what they think, adjust my speech and actions accordingly to my imagination, the consequence is that I will be punished. After reading this first story, I think you'll understand why I am who I am.

1

TRUE STORY

UNDER THE AUTUMN SUN, A LITTLE BOY CROUCHED UNDER a poplar tree, captivated by the colours in a leaf held against the light. A drop of dew slid off, catching the sun's rays as it fell to the ground. Just then, his older sister, with a smile bright as the day, ran up to him. They shared a grin, and their heads came together as they whispered about their big plan, the leaves falling gently around them.

They were always together, exploring the farm with its fields, cows, and noisy chickens. But since she started school, their adventures were now squeezed into weekends, making this day even more special. They had a secret mission—one they were determined to complete.

The sister, serious but excited, needed matches for their plan. Her brother, proud of his contribution, had already snuck a cigarette from their father's truck. He was sure their dad wouldn't notice. The sister's task was harder—she had to get the matches without their mom seeing. They were confident they could trick her, just as long as the brother created a distraction.

As the little boy pretended to show off his bike skills, falling over and over to keep their mom's attention, his sister sneaked into the house. She grabbed the matches and they raced to the barn, giggling with excitement.

But their secret didn't last. The smoke from their experiment betrayed them. When their father found them, his anger was terrifying. The boy winced as the burning cigarette was pushed against his lip. The girl's heart broke as she felt the sting of her father's slap.

She ran, tears streaming down her face, and hid by the shed. Her lip throbbed, but the real pain was in her heart. She vowed never to love again, thinking it would only lead to more hurt. As dusk fell, she wished for the comfort of her teddy bear and fell into a troubled sleep.

In her dreams, an angel appeared, glowing with warmth and kindness. The angel showed her a future where she was alone, bitter, and filled with regret because she had shut out love. The girl cried out, asking the angel to help her, to stop the hurt.

When she awoke, her father was calling her name. She stumbled into his arms, wanting to ask why he had hurt her so much, but the words wouldn't come. As he carried her back to the house, she thought she heard him say, "I'm sorry. I love you." But her heart wasn't ready to believe him—not yet.

2

WHY DO WE CARE WHAT OTHERS THINK

TODAY I REALIZE THAT THAT CHILDHOOD EXPERIENCE settled into my heart for decades. I didn't believe my father then. He's gone now, and I wonder at times why I didn't stand up more and question his actions. All I needed to say was, you hurt me. But I didn't.

I realize now that my nature was formed by fear. I feared his retaliation. Then, I feared retaliation from strangers. I didn't stand up much at all over the years.

Even those closest to me could fill me with apprehension because I had an imaginary knowing I "could" be hurt if I didn't act the way I imagined I should with others.

This is why I care about what others think of me.

CHILDHOOD TRIGGERS

Could a childhood experience create a lifelong fear of many things? Of course, it can. Ask yourself, why do you care what others think of you? What happened to trigger that fear? Because seriously, you were not born this way.

I did some research about being born with a survival instinct.

When we walked with woolly mammoths and sabre-toothed tigers, mankind was afraid of getting eaten. That survival instinct kept being reborn into modern day. It's called the need for inclusion. Particularly, group inclusion was necessary for survival. Today, our greatest predatory threat is our own species, both physically and socially.

Regardless of this threat and the need for acceptance —the fear that we won't be accepted—remains a powerful influence on our thoughts and feelings. This in large measure fuels the existential anxiety that has become the hallmark of a generation, *driving everything from people-pleasing to co-dependence to over-sharing on social media.*

LIZARD BRAIN

In other words, while our brains have evolved, that part of it that believes we must ensure we are included in our tribe, no matter the cost, is alive and well. It's commonly referred to as our lizard brain.

In *Psychology Today*, Joseph Troncale M.D. writes that the Lizard Brain refers to the oldest part of the brain, the brain stem, responsible for primitive survival instincts such as aggression and fear ("flight or fight")." The lizard brain is a physical location at the base of the brain. It's called the amygdala, and tells us we need to slow our roll and not get too far out ahead of our pack. Because without our pack to protect us, our very lives are in danger.

This part of the brain causes much of our people-pleasing tendencies. It prods us to do what everyone else is doing so we don't alienate anyone. It encourages us to hold back and not outshine others lest we are rejected.

You can see why so many of us constantly fight our fear of what others think of us. It's only human.

BUT, THERE IS GOOD NEWS.

We don't need to just throw up our hands and give up, fated to always bow to and fight those in charge. We can change our brain's pathways, making the lizard brain less prominent in our lives, decisions, and actions.

Neuroscientists have discovered that our brains are malleable. Neuroplasticity is the official term for our ability to form new connections and neural pathways in our brains by changing our reactions to daily events. How? First, by noticing what people, words, and situations trigger our lizard brain. What makes you feel unworthy? What makes you respond to going along with the crowd even when you don't want to?

For me, fear was triggered when I wanted to explore, travel, try new things, and the fear of my parents, that Dad especially, would not approve. Hell, I felt sick every time I wanted to try something new. My subconscious (that little girl experience) was alive and well. She literally ruled my adult life.

An old boyfriend of mine enjoyed toking up marijuana back in the day. I had never tried and vowed I never would. Somehow, he convinced me one evening at my parent's house. They were away visiting and I thought well, I'm home, I'm safe, sure let's have a drag of this funny smelling cigarette.

I don't know how others react, but for me, I went into an imaginary panic instantly after the first inhale. I could see lights twinkling in the distance and imagined my parents were driving into the yard. They were coming home. They would catch us. They would be disappointed and angry. I was nineteen years old.

I hid in my room, in a corner, a blanket tossed over my head and nothing could persuade me coming out. In the end, there were no car headlights in the distance. No one was coming home. I imagined the worst for myself. Later, after the drug wore off and I came back to my senses, I realized that panic was in me and that is why it could so easily be triggered. I've never done drugs since.

SIX SIGNS YOU WORRY TOO MUCH ABOUT WHAT OTHERS THINK

IF YOU READ MY BOOK, *HOW TO KEEP THE GROUND FROM SHAKING* which can be found on Amazon, I wrote that even though I enjoyed alcohol off and on over the years, I became addicted to it for three years every day, immediately after my open-heart surgery scare. I was alcohol intolerant and it made me sick. But that didn't stop me from drinking every day for those three years. I realized one of the main reasons I drank was to fit in. I thought I was stronger than that. But I wasn't. I wanted to fit in because I didn't want people to think I was different.

Not until I decided to dig deeper about why I cared so much what others thought about me, did I come to the conclusion I was living out of a subconscious fear. Actually, as much as we'd like to show that we don't care about what others think about us, we do. Some people are so preoccupied with it, they seldom take part in things they like. Whether it's the feeling of embarrassment, or the fear of being laughed at, caring too much only holds us back from what we want.

My fear of what others thought was also a fear of being emotionally and physically (I grew up with spankings) abused. I wasn't a bad girl, however, the style of discipline I grew up with, influenced my mind and body every time I participated in a variety of sports and functions.

For example, before a volleyball or fastball game as a teenager, I would have the most severe stomach cramps. Over the years, I was taken into hospital many times for fear I had appendicitis. It was always fear.

I remember the local physician telling my mother she should send me on a trip to relax. Germany was his suggestion. My mother gave him a piece of her mind at that one!

Over the years, I've learned to control and release that pain, but the stigma stands. By the way, a nice cup of tea works miracles.

Here are a few signs to know if you worry too much about what others think of you.

1. YOU WANT EVERYONE TO LIKE YOU

In an attempt to ensure everyone likes you, do you do and say things which aren't *you?* For example, me on the golf course is almost comical. I am an average to good golfer and maintain the pace well. However, if I'm with beginners, or if a team happens to come up behind, I start sweating. My palms are wet, I can't hold the golf club well, and I feel anxious. Without me even realizing, subconsciously, I am afraid the team behind will scold me for holding them up. That anxiety is worse when a Marshall drives by. They're just doing their job, monitoring the fairways. But I decide they're watching me so I don't screw up and slow the game for others. It's hell out there. And yet I'm a good golfer for pete's sake! I'm not living my authentic life, which leaves me feeling miserable. You probably can relate. When you are continuously doing or saying what *others* want, you are cheating yourself from what *you* want. It's impossible to please everyone all of the time. I love golf, but sometimes, I don't have a good time and this time, it's all in my head. What a spinning wheel of garbage thinking this is.

2. YOU CAN'T SAY NO

Whenever someone asks me for a favour, I don't just jump, I ask how high! I think it's polite to accommodate. I learned that with my mom. But underlying is that niggling little girl who thinks she's doing something wrong for not complying with others' (parents') wishes.

Do you automatically feel obliged to help those who ask you a favour? Even when that might affect your job or another aspect of your life? You have a hard time saying no because you don't want to let them down. If they feel disappointed, you worry they will stop liking you. When I worked in accounting, I would be asked to check or adjust some figures. And instead of putting it on my to do list and getting to the task when I finished what I was currently doing, I would jump and do their request and then get back to my work. Every. Single. Time.

3. YOU ARE WORRIED ABOUT WHAT YOU SAY

Social media exasperates me. I find I over think my responses. A lot of times, I don't respond because I don't want a complete stranger to think bad of me. How silly is that? They don't know me and I don't know them. Yet, I panic that I won't be seem in a kind, positive light. I've quit groups that had strong opinionated members that I felt I couldn't stand up with. Not to, but with. There were plenty of people arguing and calling each other names, and I certainly was not willing to be one of them. Do you constantly think about what you are saying, writing and your manner of speaking? Are you your worse critic, and you constantly self-censor yourself? Taking the safe route every time will make you seem like the quiet, shy type. However, you are sure to miss out on opportunities to share your opinions and ideas, and form new relationships. Sometimes I post my opinion even when asked, and then moments later delete it. I'm such a woos!

4. YOU ARE OVER-ANALYZING YOURSELF

This one kills me every time I think about it. I write. I write a lot. And even though I can create a manuscript in record time, I go back over and over and over adjusting and rewording. Even when it's been edited and ready for publication, I sweat the cover, the font sizes and sometimes hold production because I don't like something. It's a good manuscript, but I analyze my purpose for producing it in the first place. How about you? Are you constantly observing each and every one to check if anyone has noticed you falling short of expectations? Your perceived expectations, of course. More importantly, are you are trying to look at yourself from someone else's angle? The constant worrying and thinking will never let you be satisfied with the way you are and the way you do things.

5. YOU DON'T TAKE FEEDBACK WELL

I don't know if it's feedback or that my mother screeched at me, but since that day a long time ago, I've never baked a pie again. Picture this. Middle of summer, we're home from school, and the day is nice and hot. Mother has the filling and pie dough ready. She has a chore to do so she asks me to put the pie together, stick it in the oven and bake it for supper. Piece of cake—I mean pie, I think. I rolled out a chunk of pie dough and it wasn't round or perfect enough. I clumped it back tougher and rerolled it. Still not good enough. I clumped it up a second time and tried to roll it out. It fell apart. It wouldn't stick as one piece. I was devastated. Mother walks in and sees the crumbles of dough all over the table. She literally screeches, "What did you do?" I'd not heard a louder desperate voice since. I'm pretty sure she told me pie dough does not like to be re-clumped. And not in a hot kitchen. But I thought I would make it just right. I forgot the principles of dough. How about you? Even though, deep down you know that feedback is probably good for you and will actually help you excel, you just can't deal with it. Constructive criticism gets you down, which leads to you telling yourself that you are not good enough. By the way, I ran crying to my room and later when I came out, she had the pie baked. The crust was tiny pieces knitted together like a jigsaw puzzle. It looked wonderful, tasted great. But I know it was a lot of work for her to salvage the crusts.

6. YOU DON'T ASK FOR HELP

I'm the worst when it comes to asking my husband. I don't ask when I need help cleaning the house, or bringing in heavy items. But I do this with everyone. It was near Christmas and there was a great sale on a specific wine that my family enjoyed. I bought a case for the holidays and given it was shortly after my open heart surgery, I contemplated asking for help to take the case to my car. Listen folks. You'll think I'm daft. I stood there for a solid five minutes arguing with myself. I can do this. You're not supposed to lift for at least thirty days until your breast bone heals. But I can do this. Finally, I sort of compromised. I had the clerk put the case in a shopping cart and I wheeled it out and slowly shifted it into my car. I am a fool. I could have damaged myself permanently. But I'm a fool who won't ask for help because I think I don't deserve it. I think they don't like to be inconvenienced. When you are taking yourself out of your comfort zone to prove useful to others, do you feel hesitant to ask for anyone's help? Do you worry that you will be judged for not being competent or capable enough to handle things on your own? That sucks big time. I've always been a capable woman. I guess I forgot I too could ask for help.

You might be wondering why I needed open-heart surgery. I was born with a bicuspid valve on my aorta, but most people have tricuspid valves that help control blood flow through the heart. My two flaps were worn out and needed a third. Now, I'm proud to say I'm a card-carrying member of the bovine family! That extra little flap from a cow gives me confidence and hope that I'll live a long, healthy life.

4

THE BENEFITS OF NOT CARING SO MUCH

OVER THE YEARS I JUSTIFIED THAT I CARE BECAUSE IT'S helpful for other people. I forgot me in the mix. A prime example was the year three of my siblings all announced they were planning to be married. I too was recently engaged to be married however, I choose not to set a date because the others were already planning. Now you have to understand, we were four born in five years, I was the oldest and already thirty. Our parents bugged us enough why no one was getting married and suddenly, here we were. I felt bad for my dad because financially he had to pay his portion for three weddings in one year. Then the unexpected happened. Mother said to me, "Well, since we're booking a band, halls, caterers and such for three, I've set your date too." You're getting married this day because Joe the band leader and Hazel the caterer are both available."

What? Imagine my surprise. In just under a year, our family had four weddings. Financially, it must have been tough on Mom and Dad, but they seemed ready for it. After all, they had been hoping someone would get married soon. Since I was the last to tie the knot, I wanted to help.

While the others ordered fancy invitations, I made mine using a word processor, coloured paper from the dollar store, and a black-and-white printer. Instead of shopping with my mom at bridal stores like my sister, I found a nice dress around the corner, on sale for $50. Unlike the others, who had big gift-opening parties with rented halls and lavish meals, I kept mine simple, hosting it in my new home's backyard. Although we all received gifts and money, I offered mine to my dad to help cover the costs. I knew this was expensive for him, and I didn't want him to be upset. But he refused my offer. I was his first-born daughter—how could he not pay for my wedding?

He and Mom planned it. I'm being facetious, but honestly, it really bothered me. Sometimes it's healthy to listen to some people's opinions. There are people in our lives who we can trust to tell us like it is if we tell them our plans, hopes, and dreams. But sometimes it doesn't. And that's the time to stand up. But we often listen to what other random people think as much or more than those trusted advisers. My parent are trusted advisers. I listened.

Maybe you've heard something like this:

- He's not good enough for you.
- Why not get a steady job and retire with a nice pension?
- You shouldn't train so much, you'll hurt your back and legs.
- You shouldn't go to college. You'll just get married, have kids, and it'll be a waste of money.
- Don't forget where you came from.

Oh yes. These statements come from naysayers and need to be ignored. Do what you believe is right for you. Here are the benefits to listening to yourself for a change.

1. LESS STRESS

What's more stressful than wanting something so badly you can taste it, and yet hearing from everyone around that it's impossible? I finished my university degree and the last summer I had free before working, I wanted to tour Europe. In those days, I could backpack, spend very little and see a lot. My parents were devastated I would do this instead of working right away to pay off my educational debts. We were both right. But I persevered this time. The struggle it takes, the energy it takes to desire and yet resist is fierce. I trusted my own instincts and did it my way. Best time of my life. Do what you desire, because you will encounter less stress in your life. You'll experience freedom instead. A miracle happened when I returned. I had a bursary (loan to be paid back) for a portion of my education. Because I was willing to teach in a Northern territory of the province, the loan was honoured and I didn't have to pay it back financially. It was a blessing in disguise.

2. MORE JOY

When I stopped letting other people make my decisions for me, I could finally live the life I knew I was here to live. I didn't listen to my parents when they said sending me to university would be a waste of time and money. I got my degree. I followed my bliss. I waited to marry until I was thirty. And I travelled the world. I worked and I bought my own corvette. I worked and I paid off my loans quickly. The joy from listening to your heart will fill you up in unexpected ways.

3. LIVE WITH INTEGRITY

When you live with integrity, you actually influence, inspire and motivate others. That may seem strange since, like me, you may have been living in fear of making mistakes. But the opposite indeed happens. Living your authentic life, one that is in alignment with your personal values, you will experience less fear. You will experience less fear of making a mistake, having regrets, not having what you need. When we live with integrity, life becomes sweeter, and we have clarity about what we should do next.

4. COMMUNITY

Herman Hesse wrote that the only reality is the one we have inside us. What makes people's lives so artificial and unworthy is that they falsely regard outside images as reality and they never allow their own world to speak. When you change what's inside, like your beliefs and thoughts, and once you are living your purpose instead of what others think you should do, you'll meet others who share common goals and dreams. You'll experience serendipity—you'll start randomly meeting people who will further your path and who will support you on it. You'll find a feather, a coin, a sign that you're on the right track. After that, it will be much easier to let go of friendships with the naysayers in your life.

5. CONNECTIONS

When we are living our authentic truth, we naturally draw people to us. I learned this phrase decades ago and it's proven true for me over and over. When I am clear about what I want, the universe provides. Providence moves in all manner of ways and means to support me. Because what else happens is that your energy changes. People pick up on the "vibe" of others who are living their life on their own terms. It's attractive. (as in the Law of Attraction.) So instead of losing out on friendships or connections because you go ahead and do what others have told you to do, act for yourself and you'll increase your connections. They will be plentiful and deeper than you've experienced as a follower. Time to tell yourself, it just doesn't matter. Don't care. It's my life. Grab your teddy bear, turn and walk away on your path.

FIVE STEPS TO STOP PEOPLE-PLEASING

I HOPE THAT THE LIST OF BENEFITS IN THE LAST SECTION has increased your desire to make a change. I hope you're willing to look at some more options to release caring too much about others and caring more about yourself.

Sir Issac Newton's Third Law states, "For every action, there is an equal and opposite reaction."

You have to take this law seriously. Caring too much about what others think, is like a destructive action which creates a destructive reaction, and not caring about what others think is a constructive action which in turn creates a constructive reaction. Pretty simple.

PATTERNS

Let's look at some specifics. The pattern of allowing yourself to be influenced by your own imagination that others don't approve of you in one aspect of life, big or small, especially in your immediate and intimate relationships, will be present in everything else. It doesn't matter how small something is, it will be present in the largest thing that person does. You can't have a breech in a tiny thing and not expect it to show up in something massive. It reflects everywhere. Your giving your power away to a stranger on social media, gets reflected in your dealings with getting your ideal job, or meeting your soul mate or buying your first special home. It reflects in everything in your life.

Realizing this could make you take your own choices a lot more seriously. If you're not committed to making your own decisions comfortably, that lack of commitment will show up everywhere in your life.

The cool thing is that you're not stuck this way. I think this is the mistake a lot of people make. They think that once they identify the pattern and cause and effect, they think that's who they are, and they're stuck like that forever. That's not true at all. It may take a while, or you'll discover rather quickly, you are more of a caregiver than you need to be. No matter how long, there is hoping to change.

Enjoying helping the next person is a great gift and a positive trait to have, however, it should not cause you grief or misery. Keep coming on this change journey with me. Here are some more ways to stop people-pleasing and get into the habit you couldn't care less.

1. SET BOUNDARIES

People-pleasing is when you always go out of your way to satisfy someone else, at the expense of your own happiness. It's called self-illusion when in business or your personal life, there's one enemy you will come up against again and again. This enemy will make you question yourself and doubt your every move. It's like a dark force that has its teeth sunk into you. A monster that brings fear and reluctance into your life. This enemy is you.

You may have heard of the concept to set boundaries as simple as putting your hand up to stop and not let the other person get the better of you. You may also have heard that when you set up boundaries, you are helping the person more in the long run. You are being more of a support system for the person, rather than doing their work for them. But I'm suggesting you set up a boundary for your worst enemy. And you now know who that is, you. You only have one life to live, and learning to set boundaries will help you live it to the fullest. How do you set your own boundaries against yourself?

Use a mirror and take a look at your results. Take a look at your reflection that shows the habits and behaviours you display. For example, I sub- and unconsciously believed that nobody will pay for my skills, books and ideas. I didn't market my books for a long time. Or how about this example. I teach people to invest in themselves in my financial management courses and encourage them to invest their money for their long-term future. I saw in my clients that those who didn't believe that others would invest in them, didn't feel comfortable investing in themselves either. They're seeing a mirrored image of their own belief.

The boundary is take the action to right yourself before you can right anyone else.

2. LEARN TO SAY "NO"

Saying "no" is a real challenge for many people. How about you? Do you want freedom from always being at the whims of others? You have to start someplace. Notice how you feel when you are asked to do something. Maybe you are invited to an event that you don't want to attend, but feel you "should." Take a deep breath and say, "no thanks." Start out by saying "no" to small things and then work your way up to larger requests.

Not being able to say no is just a bad habit. It's a pattern that can be changed. You're not the highest version of yourself which you can imagine, you're the lowest version of yourself which you can accept. It's time to imagine yourself saying no on a regular basis. Then put it to the test next time you open the fridge door, or a colleague wants a favour, or your spouse has an idea. Practice saying no.

3. OWN YOUR OPINION

Your opinion matters because it's simply a personal power of choice. But are you uncomfortable to stand alone if others don't share your opinions? It's natural to want to fit in—actually, our brains are hard-wired with the desire to be one of the gang. Start finding times when it feels safe to share your opinion, even if no one else agrees. You may want to practice this with close friends and family first and then once you feel more comfortable, expand sharing to other groups of people, for example, at work. Now before you go ahead and expose yourself, (your opinion that is) let me caution you about the possibility you could have a Charlie Brown personality.

James Kaufman discusses the educational value of comics in his book *Teaching for Creativity in the Common Core Classroom*. He highlights how comics can be an effective tool for visual literacy development, improving reading comprehension, and fostering critical thinking skills. Kaufman emphasizes that comics can engage students in a unique way, helping them to navigate complex narratives and ideas through the interplay of text and visuals.

He writes that Charlie Brown is likened to neuroticism. He is a model neurotic. He is prone to depression and anxiety with paralyzing fits of over-analysis. Constantly worrying if he is liked or respected, he has a perpetual, usually dormant crush on the little redheaded girl, taking small joys in her foibles (like biting her pencil) that may make her more attainable. He is noted for his inability to fly a kite. But you are not Charlie Brown. You can fly your own kite. Own it.

If you are looking for more detailed information, you might want to explore Kaufman's various works or resources that discuss his approach to integrating creativity into education.

4. END JUSTIFYING

People-pleasers often feel the urge to justify their inability to do something asked of them. Do you make excuses when all you really want to say is not today? But in reality, you do not have to answer to anyone but yourself. The next time you find yourself getting ready to explain yourself and why you can't do what another person wants you to do, stop yourself. Zip it. You will usually find people don't ask for an explanation. You may be imagining they care. They don't. Just like you won't either, very soon. Tell yourself you couldn't care less what they think because you care what you think.

This reminds me of a fable shared by Vanzant about a rabbit and a witch that teaches us about the power of choice and what happens when we don't ask for what we want and what happens when we don't listen to ourselves.

The witch and the rabbit lived together in the woods, spending many days walking and talking along the forest trails. One day, the witch asked the rabbit to come with her to another town. Though the rabbit didn't want to go, he stayed silent and walked alongside her, pretending everything was fine. After a long walk, they stopped to rest. The rabbit said, "I'm so thirsty." The witch plucked a leaf from a tree, blew on it, and handed the rabbit a gourd filled with water. He drank it without saying a word. They continued on their journey.

Later, they stopped again, and the rabbit said, "I'm hungry." The witch picked up a stone, blew on it, and turned it into a bunch of radishes. The rabbit ate them quietly, and they kept going. After a while, the rabbit slipped and tumbled down a mountainside into a deep cavern. The witch transformed into a bird and flew to his side. Seeing he was badly hurt, she gathered leaves and stones, spoke a few magic words, and made a healing salve, which she rubbed on him. The witch stayed with the rabbit until he felt better. Then she turned into an eagle, lifted him, and flew him back to his nest before leaving.

Days passed, and the witch didn't see the rabbit. She searched for him, called for him, but he was nowhere to be found. One day, by chance, she bumped into him in the forest. "Why have you been hiding from me? Why didn't you let me know you were better?" she asked.

"Stay away from me!" the rabbit cried out. "I'm afraid of you! I don't like you or the magic things you do."

The witch was heartbroken. Tears welled up in her eyes as she replied, "I helped you because I thought you were my friend. You accepted my magic gifts as if you were. But now you turn against me. Don't you know I could destroy you? But I won't, because I've been your friend. Instead, I'll put a curse on you. From now on, if you don't speak your wishes, you'll lose the power to wish. And when you have no wishes and become afraid, your fears will come true."

What's the moral of the story? That which you do not choose will choose you, and that which you fear will find you.

5. TAKE SMALL STEPS

Be patient with yourself. Allow yourself time to change. Do not be hard on yourself because you have probably been a people pleaser your entire life. You may have even been taught and encouraged to be one. I know I was. I grew up kind and helpful. But I took it too far.

My husband and I lived in a little paradise on Vancouver Island far away from our roots. When my father died, my mother needed support. She didn't handle being by herself well, and her health began to fail. She became dependent on us and her body failed often. I know the power of thought, and I knew in my heart, she was convincing herself to stay sick because she wanted to be with Dad. It took a decade to get over his death. Longer actually. She couldn't see herself with him. No amount of discouraging her to think well and healthy thoughts could persuade her to change. As the oldest of the four kids and first daughter, I took the responsibility to move back from my little paradise and be my mother's official caregiver. This lasted twenty years. Was I the witch or the rabbit? A lot of both I admit.

The small steps I took were in fact, huge. We moved back thousands of miles. We began new jobs. I drove hundreds and hundreds of miles in four seasons of weather to make sure she had what she needed and took her to all her appointments. What would I do different?

Only one thing. I would have reduced the amount of time I spent caring, but I couldn't shake what she would think of me if I said no at least once a week. In retrospect, that's what I would do different. That's a small step. Say no once a week.

During that once a week time, I would do something special for myself.

How about you? Start by noticing who you defer to consistently and the feelings you experience when you feel that urge to do whatever it takes to make the other person happy. If doing the thing will make you happy too, then do it. If not, start standing up for yourself by offering a simple, "no, thanks" or "no, I can't today." That's a small step that reaps huge rewards.

6

FOUR MIND HACKS TO STOP WORRYING ABOUT WHAT OTHER PEOPLE THINK

SELF-FULFILLING PROPHECY. THIS CONCEPT HAS ROLLED through my brain for decades. In *Emerson Essays*, the chapter about Self-Reliance states:

> You must trust yourself: every heart vibrates to that iron string. Accept the place the divine Providence has found for you; the society of your contemporaries, the connection of events.

I felt her power (Providence) and was stunned by her accuracy. Each time I believed something or made a commitment to a project or situation, "stuff" would appear in the cosmos around me proving that the belief and commitment were right. Has this happened for you?

The universe is a unique special mechanism. It responds to us. You think something will happen, it likely will. Maybe not right away, but if you think about something long enough, you see it. It's faster when you believe it.

Thoughts are illusive and weird at the same time. It's natural for our brains to care about how others perceive us, it's not always healthy. How often do you find yourself creating mind stories about what someone thinks about what you just said or did? How often are you creating dissatisfaction in your life that can be turned around just by turning around your thoughts? Try these mind hacks the next time you find yourself caring too much about what someone thinks of you. Like today.

1. EVERYONE HAS FLAWS

We all make mistakes. We all have issues that we could work on to become better, happier people. And yes, that includes you, but it also includes those people you worry won't like you or don't think you are good enough. Or you're too good! I was athletic and smart. That put me in a category of being envied and disliked on teams of gals who were not necessarily as talented. I'm not friggin' bragging here. I'm just saying, there are people who do some things better than others. And you are probably one of those people who can accomplish something lickety-split that no one else can. In my experience, little did the girls who chided me know, their barbs destroyed me. How many times I would go home and cry for hours on end. They didn't know. All the power to them—all gone from me! While it's not healthy to drag up every negative thing you can think of about someone else, (said out loud to those who envied me) it's good practice to remember in general that no one is perfect. (Including me!)

2. LIFE IS SHORT

I'm seventy as of this second edition writing. Pisses me off that seven, I repeat, seven decades have flashed by. If I knew then what I know now… wishful thinking, isn't it? But those of you young and younger, know this. Time fleets so it's important to get over the shit fast! It feels good to be liked and admired. But there are bound to be people in this world that you just don't click with. It's a big pond out there. Being okay with that could be challenging, but if you find yourself trying to do everything you can to make someone like you, you are wasting your energy. Life is way too short to worry about what erroneous things people might think of you. You can't control what someone thinks. Try to grab a sunbeam and put it in your pocket. Check if it's still there. How about a wisp of wind? Stick that in your pocket. Is it there? Nope. That's how illusive a thought it. You can grab yours and change them up. But you can't grab anyone else's. To ensure you are living the life you have to the fullest, it's healthier to just shrug your shoulders if someone seems to dislike you and move on. Grab your teddy bear and walk away!

3. THEY AREN'T THINKING ABOUT YOU

If I had a plug nickel for every time I thought "they" are thinking about me, I would be a billionaire. You see, most people are caught up in their own thoughts and worries. When you come into contact with someone who seems to look down on you, it may simply be that they feel bad about themselves or a choice they just made. I've learned over the years, I'm not that interesting to most people! And eventually it stopped bothering me. They, just like you and me, are caught up in their own mental world. The reality is that most of the time, people aren't thinking about us at all, but are focused on what's going on in their own lives. They often react out of that place too, not based on what you've done or said. Okay then. Why would I be so stressed thinking I need to be or say what I believe others need to hear? What do I care so much what they think? Do I want to be a fortune teller?

4. JUST DO IT ... ANYWAY

When we have a goal—something that we really desire to see happen, we can often be kept in a state of inaction because of fear of what others will think. I mentioned earlier I could get paralyzed in inaction especially in a crowd. I also feel that angst when I'm in a large, packed store. I get overwhelmed with the product choice and literally feel every eye is on me in my inadequacy. How weird and unnecessary. You may have even experienced having a close friend tell you how irrational, unlikely or just plain crazy your actions or worse, your dream is once you finally open up and share. Remember item two above? Life is short, and we have to take a deep breath and dive in if we ever want our lives to be the way we want them to be. Don't let others determine what you can and can't do. The risk is always worth taking. I write. I have written best sellers. But I remember a time when I mentioned I was writing a book and got that rolled eye response. Seriously? I'm laughing now because this, good folks, is my lucky thirteenth book! Hah! Who's laughing now?!

7

HOW EFT REDUCED WORRYING ABOUT WHAT OTHERS THINK

EFT or Emotional Freedom Technique sometimes referred to as "tapping" is proving to be one of the most effective self-help practices available. According to Robert Callahan, in his book Tapping the Healer Within, using thought field therapy like tapping, instantly conquers your fears, anxieties and emotional distress. This seemed surprising.

It utilizes acupressure and cognitive therapy to release hidden blocks that lead to emotional, mental and physical illness and unease. The method is simple and can be done by anyone. The basic practice is done by lightly tapping with your fingertips on twelve acupuncture or meridian points. This may sound too easy to make a difference, but rest assured, it works. The proof is in the research: Medical and psychology journals have published over 100 papers on the benefits of

EFT, including clinical trial results. EFT has been found effective for clearing Post Traumatic Stress Disorder (PTSD), chronic pain, phobias, depression, anxiety disorders, and physical diseases, among others.

GET TO THE ROOT

EFT is so effective because it goes to the root of your worry and anxiety. It provides you with a way to release blocks in your subconscious that are holding you back in ways you don't even realize. Memories and the beliefs we've experienced from childhood are stored in our bodies and subconscious. Simple things like, "Ladies are always polite and hospitable" can be distorted by our child's mind and we can internalize that we always have to be nice so people will think we are always a lady. This harmed me because I was such a tomboy and wanted to run and play and climb. Ladies don't scamper up walls onto a roof of a granary, do they? I did. Does that mean I'm not a lady? Bull crap. This simple statement made by a loving parent like my own mother, for example, can become one of the sources of our deep-seated need to please other people. Your mother may not have told you that. Mine did because she didn't want me scampering all over the farm yard up and down buildings.

By using EFT, we can release those old beliefs and memories that are keeping us from living our lives to the fullest. It is a simple, free technique you can use daily to release fears and worries without the need for long-term talk therapy.

As you tap the various points along your head and shoulders, you repeat a phrase that informs your subconscious what it is that you want to release while affirming your love and acceptance of yourself. Of course, there are many different "scripts" you can use, and you should always listen to your intuition as to what script you should use each time. I learned the technique from Margaret Lynch who is quite the expert on the simplicity of tapping. One of the first examples I learned is this basic, yet extremely effective script you could use today to start letting go of your "need" to worry about what others think of you.

Here's how I do tapping. I think about what is bothering me most and condense it into a phrase or even a word.

Then I take my left hand, open and tap underneath like a karate spot of the hand. I tap this area with my right two fingers and say:

"Even though I feel _____ about ______, I deeply and completely love and accept myself."

For example, you might say:

"Even though I feel worried and nervous about what other people think of me, I deeply and completely love and accept myself."

I repeat this three times, continually tapping the karate part.

I take the word or phrase I want cleared, i.e., nervous, and go to the top of my head, right on the top of the skull, and tap the area and say, "nervous." I repeat that word two or three times while tapping: "nervous, nervous, nervous."

Next, I go to the top of the inner eyebrow. I tap again repeating the word "nervous" three times.

Then I go to the outside of my eyes on both sides of my face. I tap there and say, "nervous, nervous, nervous."

Then I go under my eyes and tap, "nervous, nervous, nervous."

Next, I go to the philtrum, the little cleft above my mouth under the nose, tap and repeat three times.

I go under the left collarbone where there is a soft spot. I rub it and say, "Nervous, nervous, nervous."

By then "nervous" is usually gone, but I go back to the top of my head and go through the process twice or sometimes three times. Then I finish with the karate chop on the left hand repeating the original phrase three times:

"Even though I feel worried about what other people

think of me, I deeply and completely love and accept myself."

It's that simple. To learn more about of how to use EFT, search online for it. Find Margaret and she will show you. Read Callahan's book, and he will heal you. There are lots of videos online that will show you exactly how to use the technique.

It's a simple but powerful tool to tap out the frustration.

8

IS SOCIAL MEDIA CAUSING MORE SOCIAL ANXIETY?

MY NEIGHBOUR DOREEN WAS MUMBLING UNDER HER breath one day while out in her garden. She was definitely frustrated about something.

"What's wrong?" I asked her.

"I'm pissed off at the newspaper!" she replied.

"What do you mean?" I smiled. Seemed an odd thing to be annoyed about.

She explained how she wanted to reduce her stress. She decided that each day she would practice staying focused in the present and quiet her mind for a few minutes each morning. She said she was told this helps. But it lasted ten minutes tops and she couldn't figure out why she couldn't stay calm longer.

I asked about her routine in the mornings. Suddenly the obvious hit her like a ton of bricks. Immediately after waking, she would grab her cell phone and surf social media. Then she would read the paper with her mega cup of coffee. Her disposition and energy levels were at distressed levels almost immediately and her objective to stay calm took longer to achieve. No wonder she lasted only a few minutes.

She was flying out of control. We talked it through and she agreed, instead, she would start the habit of meditating first thing in the morning rather than checking on the state of the world.

The next time I spoke with her, she was excited that she was able to stay in a relaxed energy for longer periods of time and take on the rest of the day with ease and calm.

Do you find it interesting that social media and print media can trigger all sorts of distress?

I know that reading news of any sort disturbs me without me even realizing. People call each other names, certainly offer words of wisdom, but then some turkey lurkey would make a rude comment even on a good feeling post.

AGE OF TECHNOLOGY

Well, we know it's the trend. It's the day and age of technology. It's the day and age of burying your nose into a smart phone device and communicate with the world. It's social media and even though it can be fun and certainly not evil, it becomes a habit of spending more time on social media than real face to face conversations. It could and does cause people to fall into the habit of needing more validation from outside sources than from within themselves. Social media is an easy way to hide. So easy, that "troll's" have a heyday attacking people like us who care too much about what their opinion are.

What are trolls? Nasty, negative people who troll the social media threads finding topics and people to abuse in short text bursts.

Truth is, some of us have a built-in need to fit in. Social scientists call this innate response Social Comparison Theory. Basically, this theory states that we determine our self-worth by comparing ourselves to others. Even though this is a natural response, when counting on validation from others or focusing solely on how we stack up to everyone else, we can become trapped in dissatisfaction.

So, social comparison is nothing new—social media did not create it. It does, however, open up our world and we now have lots more people to compare ourselves with. Instead of only trying to keep up with the Jones', we now compare the quality of our lives and our success and happiness with people all around the globe.

Studies of how Facebook and other social media outlets affect our lives can explain some of the reasons we continue to plug in on a regular basis. True Stress Management blog wrote that constant checking into social media applications is likened to multitasking. It may feel like you are getting a lot done and reading what everyone has to say, but it is associated with procrastination. This in itself is known to cause things like being late on dead-lines, to meetings, keeping appointments, and not listening to someone who is speaking. This causes more stress.

We all know people who are constantly checking their status updates and stop whatever they are doing when they hear the *ping* that they have a new notification. Many studies are showing that we are happier and mentally healthier when we access our social media less frequently.

So, what can we do to reduce our social comparison on social media? Here are a couple of suggestions.

UNPLUG

Obviously, the less time you spend on social media, the less effect this kind of social comparison will have on you. You may find you need to go cold-turkey for a week to recognize what a difference it makes. You have to realize unplugging is wise especially if you feel pressure about what to say, how to say it and to whom. Right away you will know if you are afraid of retaliation or are willing to jump in and converse with strangers. You know who you are and what you can handle. If it's stressful, unplug. Grab your teddy bear, turn around and walk away.

LIVE YOUR LIFE

When you aren't caught up in constantly checking your status updates, you'll actually live your life.

Are you one of those who stares at your phone walking? Do you try to peek while you're driving? Are you that cad who checks the phone at the dinner table? If so, it's time you took control of your reality and become more conscious of your surroundings. You wonder what total strangers think of your latest post? Stop posting. Take a break instead and live your life. You'll be more engaged in things that really matter instead of wishing you had the perfect life like so-and-so or so-and-so and especially like so-and-so.

SCHEDULE SOCIAL MEDIA TIME

Dr. Pamela Rutledge discusses the question, "Are you wasting too much time using Facebook or Twitter?" in her article on *Psychology Today* titled "The Pressures of Social Media: Should I Disconnect?" In this article, she emphasizes the importance of social media mindfulness, encouraging readers to reflect on how and why they use social media and to consider whether it's supporting or hindering their goals. She advises that if you find yourself spending too much time on platforms like Facebook or Twitter, it may be time to limit your use or even quit the platform.

Can you answer this honestly? Are you wasting time? Is your life focused on what others are saying instead of taking stock of your own surroundings? Sure, it's easy to get sucked into Facebook-land. So that you don't waste your life in front of your computer, set aside ten to fifteen minutes a day to participate in social media. Finally, consider "unfriending" those people who seem to trigger your social comparison negatively the most. Recognize that whatever you do, it is a question of you making choices, not the mysterious power of social media. Stop giving away your power to social media.

9

FIVE THINGS TO REMEMBER TO IMPROVE YOUR SELF-ESTEEM

ARE YOU OVERLY CONCERNED ABOUT WHAT OTHER PEOPLE think about you? Do you find yourself worrying about what others say about you? Are you in constant fear? Listen, it's normal to feel uncertain and some apprehension at times. But that triggers more thoughts about what's wrong about yourself. And that's the culprit that enhances fear rather than improves on your current being.

Fear motivates more anxiety, distrust, cowardice, insecurity, uncertainty, worry and a need to escape. Is that how you want to live out your life? I have believed for quite some time that I create my reality. When I choose to believe my fear is real—I suffer, and what I know for sure, fear is not real. It's my "perception" of a situation that is real. Fear is the energy I plug into it. While it is natural to seek the approval of others, those who have a high self-esteem, and are self-confident, are able to discount the negative opinions of others and to remain assured of their own self-worth.

Focusing on building your self-confidence can be made easier when you keep these five things in mind the next time you find yourself worried about what someone else believes about you. How does one do that? A key component is to choose to change perception. For example, if you don't like what you read, (in newspapers, on social media) or see on television, we go into resistance and want to change it. But can you? Can you change something from your comfy couch when you see it on television? Ninety-nine percent of the time, no. But you can change how you react or don't react to the situations.

1. NEVER GUESS WHAT OTHERS MIGHT BE THINKING

You are not a crystal ball reader. Maybe you are, and if that's the case, you probably don't worry too much about what others think. You are not a fortune teller. Or are you? We fool ourselves when we think we know what someone else is thinking. Oh sure, you can feel tension and read energy to a degree. But to actually know what someone else is thinking is poor judgment. You cause yourself much unnecessary suffering when you waste your energy imagining that others may intend you harm. You truly have no idea what anyone else is thinking. Train yourself to avoid making any assumptions about what others may be thinking—and train yourself to avoid making any assumptions about why other people choose to do or to say something—or to not do or not say anything.

2. LIVE YOUR OWN LIFE

Certainly, when you were young, what your parents or caregivers taught you was important. You needed to learn some basics to life skills. But remember, there is no way your life is "supposed" to be lived. There are no "authorities" appointed to judge the worthiness of your life. You have no responsibility to please anyone other than yourself. Be of service to humanity, but never be anyone's doormat. Live your own life full out. Live boldly with vision, purpose, and commitment. Establish your own life purpose, and live your own life.

3. MAKE YOUR OWN CHOICES

Your plan for your life is the only plan that matters. Your parents and your family, perhaps your church and your friends, have plans for your life, but those people are mere spectators of your life—the life you get to live every day. If you're in a relationship, there's such a commodity as compromise. But if the decisions lead to discomfort, something has to be faced and changed.

4. VALUE YOUR OWN OPINIONS

Why would you consider someone else's opinions, or wishes, to be more important than your own? In fact, why should anyone else's opinions carry any weight whatsoever in how you live your life? Make your life choices sincerely and deliberately. Then never second-guess your own values and choices simply because they may not be approved of by those around you.

5. CHOOSE TO ASSOCIATE MOSTLY WITH POSITIVE PEOPLE WHO SUPPORT YOU

You can't completely avoid negative people—there are probably a few negative people in your extended family and where you work. However, you can make the choice to limit your exposure to negative people, and to cultivate friends and acquaintances who have a positive outlook on life, who share many of your essential values, and who value you as a person. Besides, it gets easier and easier to turn around and take your own path. Try it.

I love this summation quote from Abraham, by Esther Hicks:

"Your world is pointing toward an insistence on conformity which is causing you enormous grief. It's what's at the heart of all of your religious battles, and religious battles are what are at the heart of all of your battles. In other words, all of your wars and global irritation with one another are over your determination to promote sameness. Your democracy insists that it's the only government that works. And every religion (it's interesting to note) proclaims that it is the only one that works.

— EXCERPTED FROM KANSAS CITY, MO
ON 9/15/04

Value your opinions. Make your own choices. Associate with those who you feel good in their presence. And never guess what someone may be thinking. We are each unique and that's key to live out. You are a valued unique individual. Celebrate that.

CONCLUSION – THE MAGIC FORMULA

THE SECRET — A SIMPLE ONE — MAY BE A SURPRISE TO you when I share this. I'm suggesting that to finally once and for all stop caring so much about what others think, is to stop resisting or pushing back toward that which you feel is pushing on you — caring what others think.

Confused? How about this. Resistance or pushing back, is when we haven't decided whether to do something or not, but we are doing it anyway, and it's difficult. For many reasons, we may have picked up in childhood or out of the blue, those stories we tell ourselves over and over continue to perpetuate this feeling of shame that we exist at all.

The stories we tell ourselves about the facts will give us a rich experience or a poor one. The choice is always there for us to make. We cannot "tell it like it is." We can only tell it the way we choose to tell it: as a victim, as the victor, as learner, as a lover, or whatever we choose to identify with.

You will never change from one perspective to another unless there's an alternative perspective to latch onto. You might choose to stay in fear of what others say, or you might wish to replace it with a feeling of courageousness and acceptance.

ATTITUDE TRIGGERS FLASHES OF INSIGHT

One of the best ways to arouse the wish to care less is to realize that the magic of flashes of insight changes our perception of the world.

What triggers insight? Attitude!

Attitude is simply a conscious choice that drives your physical learning and behaviors. For example, you can choose to follow up on opportunities and you can choose not to. When you tell yourself not to follow up because:

- You don't want to seem pushy;
- You're too busy;
- It's too hard to get dressed and go out;
- You're not sure what to say;
- You're afraid of getting rejected.

It's the attitude that takes over.

In a study done by the Harvard Business School, results showed that top salespeople and producers:

- Don't take "no" personally;
- Accept 100% responsibility for their results;
- They don't blame the economy, competition, product;
- They spend the bulk of their time on priorities;
- They put themselves in their customers' shoes;
- Are self-disciplined and persistent;
- Are honest with themselves and the customer;
- And don't care what others think!

How many of the above elements could you relate to?

Now it's time to examine your old notions and bring awareness to them. Awareness may be all you need to dissolve an old pattern or belief.

First, ask yourself, why would you want to heal them?

If you're struggling to make basic ends meet, you might want to heal a pattern that keeps you from earning more or spending less.

If you're constantly fighting with the very person

you love, you might want to heal a pattern that keeps you from enjoying their company.

If you're sick and tired, you might want to heal a pattern that keeps you from being healthy and vibrant.

If you're constantly feeling dragged down by the opinion of others, you do want to heal a pattern that keeps you from moving forward with peace of mind.

Write a list of old fears and beliefs.

Now examine this list and decide if they are true for you right now.

Replace any of these with positive statements or affirmations that resonate as true for you. For example, if you've been repeating "I'm a failure at everything!" replace it with "I am successful in these areas in my life (fill in the blank)."

Or you tell yourself, "Nobody loves, everybody hates me!" replace it with "I don't care if they don't agree with me. I love myself!"

With each item you become aware of, ask yourself how true are your thoughts right now. It's time to look at that belief and decide once and for all if it's serving you or hindering you. It can be that simple.

I offer dozens more strategies and tips to reduce and erase fears in my book, *The Most Powerful Person on Earth!* You can find it on my website Shop Books along with other works.

My hope is you gained some flashes of insight in this

book. While the flash may arrive out of the blue, the treasure only comes when we have carefully and persistently prepared the way for it. Remember this old adage, "How do you eat an elephant?" (that is if you wanted to) "One tiny bit at a time."

Taking steps to dissolve the fear of what others might think can be arduous and overwhelming. Tacking little fears with small steps creates magic. Then the ripple effect is powerful when we are more prepared to tackle the bigger fears.

STACKED BRICK WALL

In one of my self-help programs, I share that your woes are like a stacked brick wall. If you take a brick or two out from the bottom (where the more solidly believed fears sit) the ones layered on top begin to wobble and collapse. The wall falls even if you just pulled out a couple. The essence of experience is change, and the ultimate certainty of life is that there is change and change is uncomfortable. Find the courage to change may be your greatest lesson. Use your fear to get stronger rather than run in fear.

And most of all, enjoy the process—life is a journey not a destination. Grab your teddy bear, love yourself, turn around and go your own path.

ABOUT THE AUTHOR

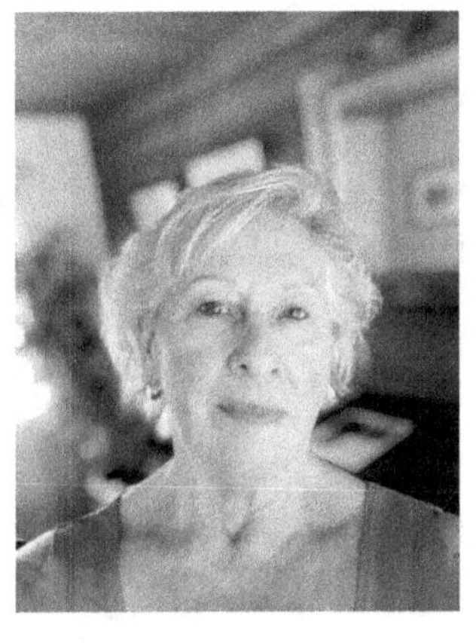

Patricia Ogilvie, MEd. Freelance Copywriter and Editor.

Her experience and qualifications include the following:

Trained in Advanced Level Direct Response Copy Writing — American Writers and Artists Institute,

Former **Systems Analyst** known for intense research, analysis and attention to detail,

Stays current on new advertising trends for different products and services,

Thorough understanding of *The Chicago Manual of Style* (CMOS) for grammatical structure,

National Member, **Canadian Association of Professional Speakers.**

Patricia is married to Randy and lives in Alberta Beach, near Edmonton, Alberta. Edmonton is the city boasting the world's largest Shopping Mall in the only debt-free province in Canada. Ironic analogy, isn't it?

She's been a professional copywriter, editor and speaker for over fifteen years, and has written fiction, non-fiction, poetry, numerous e-books as well as distance learning courses, multimedia CD's and scripts.

She is the author of three books of poetry, three successful business e-books, is the co-author of *Expert Women Who Speak...Speak Out!* a Canadian best-seller. She has written her own autobiography *The Day The Pigs Ate My Baby Brother*, which tells of her hilarious experiences growing up on a farm in the Boyle, Alberta area.

She's also written innumerable articles and short stories, not to mention adverts, training materials, press releases and more.

This is her nineteenth book.

YOUR ACTION PLAN

Contact Patricia at the social media links below or go to her website:

https://proriskenterprises.com

and tell her that you want content written, edited, or proofread.

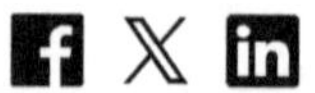

MORE BOOKS BY PATRICIA OGILVIE

If you like this book, you'll love the 1st, 2nd, 3rd, and 4th inspirational adult colouring books in my series of stress reducer and fun increasers.

Look for *Bag lady, Marbles, and Radical Self-Respect,* and the public favourite, *Life Lessons for Women* on my website www.proriskenterprises.com

HERE ARE MORE BOOKS AVAILABLE:

The Adventures of Isla 2024

The Prodigy 2023

Amazon Best-Seller: Wild Mind: Remembering Last Week's Notes Today 2017

The Most Powerful Person on Earth 2017

Believe in Magic 2016

Good Better Best 2016 Children's book

How to Keep the Ground from Shaking 2017

How to Be the BOSS of Your Own Money 2017

Find all these and more at www.proriskenterprises.com/shop

And please do leave a comment on Amazon for me. I would

love to hear your experience and how you've found releasing the fear of what others think. Appreciate you! Patricia